Heal Chagas Disease

(American trypanosomiasis)

By

Dr. Elliott Charles

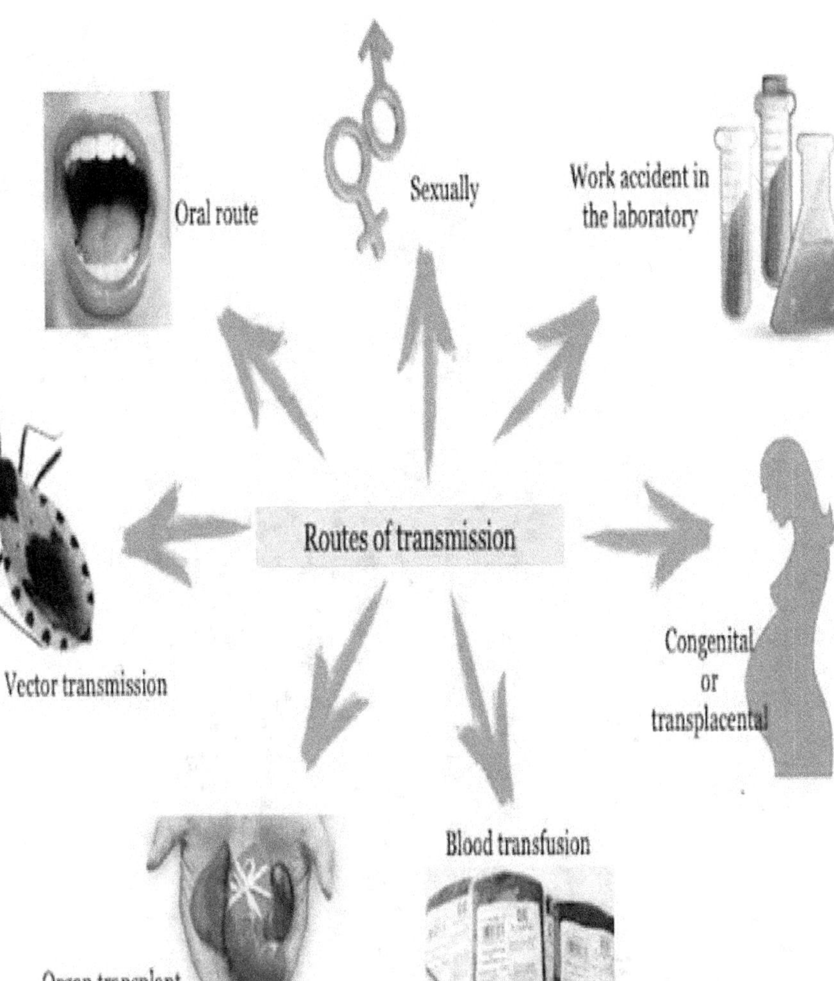

Oral route
Sexually
Work accident in the laboratory
Vector transmission
Routes of transmission
Congenital or transplacental
Organ transplant
Blood transfusion

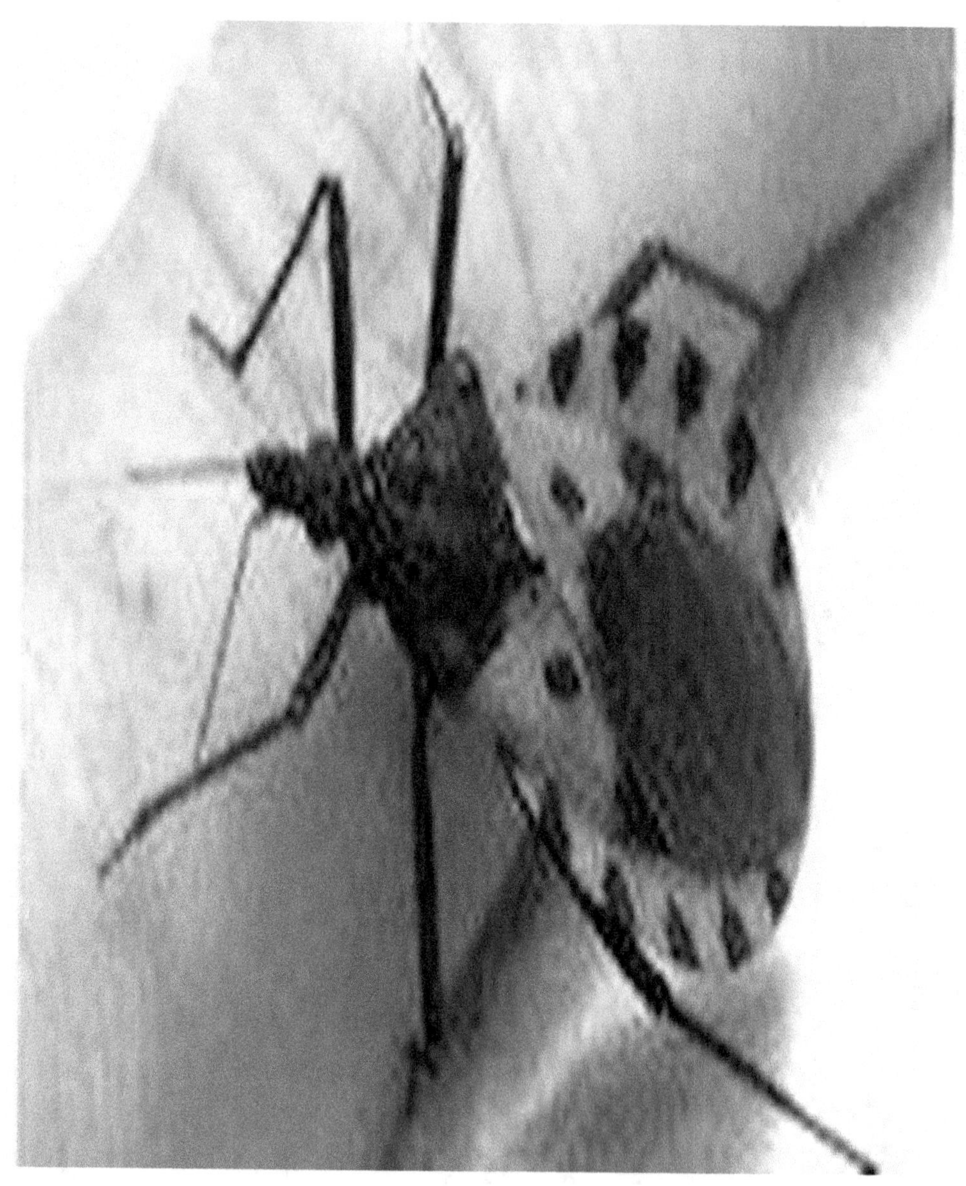

Table Of Contents

Introduction

With around 8 million chronically infected people, trypanosoma cruzi, the organism that causes Chagas disease, is a severe health concern in Latin America. Chagas disease has recently emerged as a potential public health issue in developed nations as a result of greater human travel, with considerable increases in the number of confirmed cases recorded in the United States, Canada, Europe, Japan, and Australia. Metacyclic trypomastigotes are often expelled with the feces of infected triatomines after their blood meal and enter the human host through damaged skin or healthy mucosa. Oral, congenital, blood transfusion/organ transplant, and congenital infections are additional infection pathways that may exist. In vertebrate hosts, T. coxi can be found as both amastigotes, the internal replicative form, and extracellular trypomastigotes, which freely circulate in the blood and tissues. This is understandable since T. cruzi is an obligate intracellular parasite. A self-limiting acute phase of infection that is frequently experienced by infected individuals is marked by patent (or subpatent) parasitemia. The parasites are already actively replicating in a wide variety of cell types, including macrophages, cardiac, smooth, and striated muscle cells, adipocytes, and cells of the brain and spinal cord.

While the acute stage of the illness only affects a small proportion of patients, the development of the adaptive immune response typically leads to non-sterile control of the T. cruzi infection. Those who have the illness

The host will continue to exist and maintain a dynamic equilibrium with the parasite if the parasite is not completely eradicated, which could result in a range of clinical outcomes. Because of this, while many people with long-term illness continue to be asymptomatic, 30 to 40 % of them eventually develop cardiac or digestive symptoms, such as cardiomyopathy, which can result in mega syndromes of the esophagus or colon, congestive heart failure, arrhythmia, and ultimately patient death. Even without parasites, these pathogenic changes cannot be reversed. Mice that are infected with T. cruzi for a long time develop chronic myocardial lesions that resemble chagasic myocarditis in humans.

Chapter 1

Knowing The Basics Information About Chagas Disease

What is Chagas disease exactly?

The parasite that causes Chagas disease is called Trypanosoma cruzi. The infection known as Chagas disease is also referred to as American trypanosomiasis. The parasite can infect people and animals through a variety of different channels. The most frequent cause is an insect bite. It is believed that vectors carry the Chagas illness. An "insect vector" is any insect that spreads disease (vector-borne diseases) by circulating parasites in the host's blood. 4) A kind of Triatomine bug, also known as "kissing bug," can spread the parasite that causes Chagas disease infections." Because of their propensity to pounce on people's faces, particularly around the eyes and mouth, kissing bugs came to be known by this name. T. cruzi parasites enter the host (the person or animal that has been bitten) via the bloodstream or the organs, causing damage and dysfunction that can sometimes be very serious.

Up to 8 million people in Mexico, Central America, and South America are thought to be infected with Chagas disease, the majority of whom are not aware of it. An infection can be fatal if untreated for the rest of one's life.

Effects of the Chagas disease

The effects of Chagas disease go well beyond the rural areas of Latin America where the disease is spread by insects as vectors. Large-scale migrations from rural to urban regions in South America and other parts of the world have altered the epidemiology of Chagas disease. In the United States and other areas where Chagas disease is currently present but not endemic, control methods should concentrate on limiting transmission from blood transfusions, organ transplants, and mother-to-child transfer (congenital transmission).

How does Chagas disease spread?

The disease can be contracted in a variety of ways. In regions where Chagas disease is prevalent, vector-borne transmission is the most common method of transmission. The vector insects are triatomine bugs. These blood-sucking bugs contract T. cruzi by biting an infected animal or person. Once infected, bugs spread the parasites through their feces. Houses constructed of palm thatch, mud, adobe, straw, and other materials are home to the bugs. During the day, the bugs hide in the roof and wall cracks. When people are sleeping, the bugs show up at night. Due to their propensity to nip people in the face, triatomine bugs are also known as "kissing bugs." After they bite and consume blood, they poop on the person. The person may become infected if the T. cruzi parasites in the bug feces enter the body through the skin or mucous membranes. It's possible that the sleeping, unaware individual will accidentally rub or scratch the feces into the bite wound, eyes, or mouth.

Additionally, congenital transmission occurs when an infection is transmitted from a pregnant woman to her unborn child.

blood transfusions;

Organ transplantation;

eating raw food that has been contaminated with infected triatomine bug poop; and accidental laboratory exposure It is generally accepted that breastfeeding is safe even if the mother has Chagas disease. If, on the other hand, there is blood in the milk or if the mother has cracked her nipples, she should pump it out and throw it away until the nipples heal and the bleeding stops.

Chagas disease, in contrast to the common cold and flu, does not spread through direct contact with infected animals or people.

If I have Chagas disease, should my family members be tested for the infection?

Possibly. They should be tested if:

could have contracted the disease in the same way as you did, via vector-borne transmission, for example;

Are your children, who were born following your infection; or if there are any additional clues that they might have Chagas disease.

Where in the world does Chagas disease affect?
Worldwide, Chagas disease sufferers can be found. In the Americas, however, kissing bugs are the only vector-borne method of disease transmission. The majority of people who developed Chagas disease did so in rural areas of Mexico, Central America,

and South America. In some regions of Latin America, programs to eradicate kissing bugs also known as vector control programs have stopped the spread of this disease. There is no vector-borne disease transmission in the Caribbean, including Puerto Rico and Cuba. A few isolated cases of Chagas disease caused by vectors have occurred in the southern United States.

What symptoms and indicators are present in Chagas disease?
Most of the clinical information about Chagas disease comes from people who contracted the illness as children through contact with triatomines. The severity and course of an infection can be affected by the age at which an individual became infected, the method by which the infection was acquired, or the particular strain of the T. cruzi parasite.

There are two stages of Chagas disease: the phases, both short-term and long-term. Both phases have the potential to be fatal or without symptoms.

The Romaa sign, or swelling of the child's eyelid, is a sign of acute Chagas disease. Trypanosoma cruzi can infect the eyelid and cause swelling when bug feces are accidentally rubbed into the child's eye, or when the bite wound was on the same side of the child's face as the swelling. Credit: WHO/TDR's acute phase: During this phase, which lasts for the first few weeks or months of the infection, a person may experience no symptoms or mild ones such as fever, fatigue, body aches, headache, rash, loss of appetite, diarrhea, and vomiting. Because these symptoms are similar to those of other illnesses, the majority of people are unaware that they are infected with the T. cruzi parasite.

Swollen glands, mild liver or spleen enlargement, or chagoma-like swelling at the bite site, where the parasite entered the body, may be additional signs of infection that a doctor can detect. Swelling of the eyelids on the side of the face near the bite wound or where the bug poop was accidentally rubbed into the eye is known as Roma's sign in individuals with acute phase infections. A person typically recovers within a few weeks or months, even if they experience symptoms during the acute phase. However, if the individual does not take antiparasitic medication, the infection will remain in the body. The severe infections of the heart muscle and brain known as myocarditis and meningoencephalitis rarely (less than 5%) result in the death of young children. The severe acute phase can also occur in individuals with weakened immune systems, such as HIV infection patients or chemotherapy patients.

Phase of a continuum: During this phase, which can last for decades or even their entire lives, the majority of people do not experience any symptoms. Between 20% and 30% of people infected experience heart complications, such as an enlarged heart, heart failure, altered heart rate or rhythm, or cardiac arrest (sudden death). and/or issues with the stomach and intestines, such as a megaesophagus or megacolon, that make it difficult to eat or use the bathroom.

What should I do if I think I have Chagas disease?

You should discuss your concerns with your doctor or nurse, who will examine you and inquire about your health and previous residences. Chagas disease is diagnosed with blood tests. Even if you are in good health, you should get an electrocardiogram (heart tracing test) if you have Chagas disease. You might be referred to a specialist to have additional tests and treatments done.

How is the Chagas disease managed?

There are two kinds of therapy that could save lives: treatment for the parasite's removal; and treatment for the symptoms to control the signs and symptoms of the infection.

Treatment for parasites works best early in the infection's course, but not just in acute cases. In the United States, there are two types of treatments available. The use of benznidazole in children between the ages of 2 and 12 has been approved by the FDA; It is available for purchase at is commercially available for pharmacies to purchase from a number of drug wholesalers and has been approved by the FDA for use in the treatment of children as young as 18 years old. The CDC staff can talk to your doctor about whether and how you should be treated. During treatment, most people do not require hospitalization.

I intend to travel to a rural region of Latin America where Chagas disease might be present.

How can I avoid getting this infection?

At this time, there are neither vaccines or drugs available to prevent infection. Travelers who sleep indoors in well-built facilities, such as air-conditioned or screened hotel rooms, are less likely to come into contact with infected triatomine bugs, which typically inhabit low-quality housing and are most active at night. Spraying infested homes with long-lasting insecticides, using bed nets treated with long-lasting insecticides, dressing in protective clothing, and applying insect repellent to skin that is exposed are all preventative measures. Salads, raw vegetables, unpeeled fruits, and fruit juices that have not been pasteurized should not be consumed by travelers.

Easily Means Of Contacting Chagas Disease

A triatomine bug infected with Chagas disease spreads the disease through its feces. Occasionally, this flaw is referred to as:

"kissing bug" because it can bite you in the mouth; "reduviid bug"; "assassin bug"; and "triatomine bug" because it usually bites at night. The bug excretes its feces close to where it bit. It is possible to accidentally rub the feces into the bite when you touch it

.

The feces can also accidentally be rubbed into:
a cut or open wound in your eyes, nose, or mouth If the feces are from a triatomine bug that is infected, you will be exposed to the disease.

Chagas disease can also be spread through:
by means of contamination:
blood products (transfusions); organ transplants from an infected mother to her unborn child during pregnancy and delivery; food or beverages contaminated with infected triatomine feces; laboratory accidents, such as accidental blood exposure;
needle prick injuries caused by scalpels, broken glass, and other surgical instruments

Chapter 2

Prevent And Reverse Techniques For Chagas Disease

(American trypanosomiasis) Leavell and Clark defined primary, secondary, and tertiary levels of human health prevention in a 1953 classical textbook. Depending on the disease's natural history, each one includes different methods of treatment.

Chagas disease primary defense

Primary Prevention These methods aim to prevent the disease from spreading, including the spread of new infections. Primary preventative measures make up the majority of population-based health promotion activities.

Additional Prevention

The goal of secondary prevention is to detect and address a disease in its infancy, before it significantly increases morbidity.

Third-Level Prevention

Third-Level Prevention By restoring function and reducing the amount of complications brought on by the disease, these treatments seek to decrease the impact of an already present condition.

Throughout the past few decades, the WONCA International Classification Committee has adopted Jamoulle's fourth concept, quaternary prevention. Due of this, "quaternary prevention" refers to a series of health initiatives intended to mitigate or completely avoid the adverse impacts of excessive or insufficient health system interventions.

The Quality Standards Subcommittee or Clinical Affairs Committee of the Infectious Diseases Society of America (IDSA) addressed both the strength of the recommendations and the quality of the evidence that backed them.

Strength of the Recommendation

•The recommendation for use is supported by substantial clinical benefits and robust evidence of efficacy. It ought to always be provided.

•Use recommendation is supported by moderate or strong evidence of efficacy with limited clinical benefit. It should always be available.

• There is insufficient evidence of efficacy to recommend its use or not. Or, the evidence of efficacy may not outweigh the treatment's cost or negative effects (such as drug toxicity or drug interactions): optional.

•A recommendation against use is supported by moderate evidence of an adverse outcome or lack of efficacy. In general, it shouldn't be offered.

(•A recommendation against use is supported by strong evidence of an adverse outcome or lack of efficacy. It shouldn't ever be given out.
Role of Etiological Treatment against T. cruzi Infection on Several Levels of Prevention in Public Health

Type I of Evidence to Back Up the Recommendation: evidence from at least one randomized, controlled trial that was designed correctly.
Class II: evidence from at least one well-designed clinical trial without randomization, multiple time-series studies, cohort or case-controlled analytic studies (preferably from more than one center), or significant outcomes from uncontrolled experiments.

Third type: evidence from reports of expert committees, descriptive studies, or opinions from reputable authorities based on clinical experience.

Recommendations for Therapy
Over the past few years, a number of papers and guidelines have been published that support the idea that etiological treatment is an effective intervention for both individual and public health. I will talk

about this measures applied in various situations as follows

Treatment Ideas and Strength of Evidence

A few papers and rules have been distributed somewhat recently supporting with various degrees of solidarity that etiological treatment is a successful mediation on both the individual and general wellbeing. These studies provided strength of recommendations (A), (B), and (C) at levels of evidence ranging from I to III. We discuss how these criteria were applied in various scenarios as follows.

Treatment's Success in the Acute

Phase of an Infection Several studies with evidence of Type I or II have demonstrated the beneficial effects of treatment utilizing both benznidazole and nifurtimox during the acute phase. The parasitemia, whether direct or indirect (parasitological test or molecular test), becomes negative a few days after the end of treatment, making it easy to determine whether or not a patient's treatment was effective. In addition, antibodies completely disappear (seronegativity) in at least 65% of cases, with some studies demonstrating seronegativity in 100% of cases after 18 months of treatment follow-up. Patients of all ages, from infants (congenital transmission) to adults, are affected in the same way. The reduction of antibodies always occurs prior to the absence of parasitemia as demonstrated by direct methods like Strout or the micromethod.

During the acute phase, treatment is generally well tolerated, and the reduction in clinical manifestations and even the risk of death associated with the acute phase of Chagas infection outweighs the risk of potential adverse events. All patients in the acute phase of an infection or reactivating a chronic infection must be treated, according to a strong recommendation.

Treatment Success in Unique Situations

Type III Evidence suggests that medical professionals, researchers, and others who come into contact with infected blood should be treated according to specific protocols. Existing studies (evidence Type II) have demonstrated that immunocompromised patients recover from severe reactivation manifestations like meningoencephalitis, myocarditis, and panniculitis following etiological treatment. Due to the limited ability to interpret the results of serological tests in immunosuppressed states, recovery from life-threatening acute events is the primary goal in these instances, not sero negativization. There is general agreement that these patients must be treated due to the association between the severity of reactivation and the risk of death (strength of recommendation (A)). However, there is currently no evidence to suggest that immunocompromised patients with a chronic chagasic infection without evidence of reactivation should receive etiological treatment as a preventative measure.

Treatment with benznidazole or nifurtimox is currently not recommended for pregnant women (absolute contraindication), despite the fact that some studies have reported that the etiologic treatment does not have any adverse effects on the newborn. Consistency and Tolerance Patients must be under constant medical observation during their treatment. Patients with severe acute or chronic liver or kidney disease not related to T. cruzi infection (relative contraindication) and lactating (relative contraindication) are additional contraindications to the use of etiological treatment. Patients have not reported experiencing any serious side effects, and treatment tolerance is high based on previous experiences. Although there have been instances of severe side effects, they have generally associated with difficulties in obtaining appropriate medical care or seeking timely medical attention. Adolescents and adults experience side effects more frequently than infants and children. Tolerance is high in newborns and children under the age of four. When the dosage was reduced or the treatment was stopped, there were no more side effects in any of the cases. The types of side effects that occur during treatment and their distribution are shown.

Chapter 3

Adverse Effects of Nifurtimox With Benznidazole Over Time

The usage of benznidazole and nifurtimox can also result in reversible clastogenesis and mutagenesis, which have no negative side effects. However, neither of these things have ever been proven in a general population of infected patients who are receiving treatment nor have they ever been a factor in animal models. There have been reports of toxicity against other tissues or an increased risk of lymphomas in experimental animals. It is essential to effectively control adverse effects while using trypanocidal drugs in order to administer treatment and allay unwarranted anxieties.

In the fight against T. cruzi infections, the recommendations of etiological treatment enable action on a variety of different levels of public health prevention.

Research that has been located offer proof that programs in a lot of nations can be controlled through health care tactics. More patients could receive a diagnosis, a cure, and treatment as a result, opening up a new possibility for future illness burden reduction.

Primary Prevention Level:
When treating children and young people, etiological treatment may have an indirect effect if the goal is to avoid getting a new infection. Recommendation (B) and evidence of Type III indicate that eradicating T. cruzi would prevent future congenital T. cruzi transmission to newborns in children and women who are still in reproductive age. By treating those who are infected, there will also be more people willing to donate blood and organs. Sadly, the efficacy of etiological treatment for these primary prevention indications is still unknown, but it is reasonable to assume that it is at

least equivalent to the sero negativization rates observed in the studies that are available. The development of a treatment that can be given to pregnant women, like the HIV treatment, to prevent congenital transmission during pregnancy would be another strategy. However, this strategy would require safety information on these drugs, which is currently unavailable.

An additional indication for primary prevention could be etiological treatment in the event of an accident involving material contaminated with parasites or blood samples from patients infected with T. cruzi. Since infections cannot be avoided, the treatment is not strictly a prophylaxis; however, with prompt treatment to obtain an appropriate concentration of specific drugs (recommendation (B) and evidence III), infections can be prevented immediately following accidents.

Secondary Prevention Level

If preventative measures fail to prevent infection in children, etiological treatment can still be used to treat infected children. When these children do not have significant damage from cardiac or digestive disease, etiological treatment is recommended. This is the best time to get strep and stay healthy, maintaining social, mental, and physical well-being into adulthood.

Several nations in Latin America have gradually implemented a national control program. It has included the routine screening of child populations to provide opportunities for diagnosis and treatment (recommendation (A) and evidence Type I) as well as prompt diagnosis and treatment of children born with congenital infections (recommendation (A) and evidence Type II). In order to evaluate the usefulness of serology as an indicator of the action against the vector, the positive effect of curing children detected by serological screening must be evaluated by taking into account patterns of disease transmission, evolution, and a calculation of the burden of disease attributable to Chagas disease.

The prevention of the reactivation of a chronic infection is an additional use for etiological treatment in secondary prevention. HIV/AIDS or immunosuppressive therapies put patients with chronic infections at greater risk of reactivation. It is necessary to gather evidence to determine whether preventive treatment is effective in patients with abnormal immunological parameters and no clinical reactivation signs, despite the fact that the effectiveness of etiological treatment for the clinical control of reactivation episodes has been demonstrated. In this regard, in order to lessen the likelihood of transmission through transplant, some protocols call for the treatment of organ donors who are infected with T. cruzi. In light of recommendation (A) and evidence (Type II), the treatment ought to be regarded as an act of primary prevention.

Tertiary Prevention Level
Two randomized clinical trials are evaluating the efficacy of etiological treatment for T. cruzi infection in patients with cardiac disease to reduce the negative effects of established disease. The effectiveness of benznidazole in halting the progression of cardiac disease is the subject of these trials.

Several observational studies have been published that show how etiological treatment prevents the progression of chronic chagasic cardiomyopathy in T. cruzi-infected patients. Strength of recommendation (B) and (C) were provided by these studies, which reached quality of evidence Type II. Patients with heart failure or advanced stages of

Chagas' cardiomyopathy have a poor prognosis, just like those with other causes of heart failure. It is critical to identify early factors that are determinants of disease progression due to the chronic nature of the condition and the progressive nature of heart damage. In the Chagas' cardiomyopathy physiopathology model, etiological treatment ought to be taken into consideration as a protective factor.

As previously stated, the recovery of severe reactivation manifestations like meningoencephalitis, myocarditis, and panniculitis demonstrates the efficacy of etiological treatment for controlling reactivation episodes.

In this book, it is important to consider the available evidence about etiological treatment and to maintain the perspective of etiological treatment as a public health tool in multiple levels of prevention, in addition to other interventions that are available for

Phase 1 of the control and treatment of Chagas illness

Discussion The emphasis on patient care in the primary healthcare system, the utilization of other levels of care when necessary, and the integration of psychological factors into care are recommendations for providing patients with adequate care that is on the rise.

control of vectors,

The most successful primary prevention strategies for Chagas disease are those focused on surveillance and the regulation of blood and organ donors. Nevertheless, etiological treatment is an important feature of efforts to control Chagas disease and is important for primary prevention.

Controlling congenital transmission and diagnosing infection in children (defined as chronic recent infection) or young adult patients in chronic phase without clinical manifestations (sign and/or symptom) are the best examples of secondary prevention in Chagas disease. When used in conjunction with complementary medicines in cardiac illness, the use of etiological treatment for tertiary prevention in Chagas disease is now supported by recommendation levels (B) and patients to reduce the clinical progression of the disease. For instance, cardiac transplantation is a procedure that has been used on some patients with terminal heart failure and has demonstrated clinical benefit. Stem cell transplant is a new treatment for patients in the final stages of congestive heart failure to produce cardiac regeneration by distinguishing or increasing heart myocytes or neovascular proliferation. However, the results on Chagas disease are still insufficient, and there is no consensus regarding its efficacy.

A national policy of etiological treatment of infected individuals ought to be considered an activity in relation to quaternary prevention. In recent decades, a number of nations in Latin America have utilized this strategy.

In order to properly evaluate the results and evaluate the effect of treatment on T. cruzi infection, one must have a clear understanding of the variables' combination. The tools used as indicators (parasitological, molecular, and serological tests), the stage of infection (acute or chronic) the patient was in when he or she was treated, and the time between treatment and the application of the test to assess efficacy or failure are, among other things, the main variables.

The detection of free parasites in the patient's blood or tissues, which enables clear observation of treatment failure, is the best method for determining a patient's response to a particular treatment.

The effectiveness of a treatment can only be evaluated using a small number of techniques. After a full course of treatment has been administered during the chronic phase, it is also necessary to validate new tools to promptly confirm cure or failure. Studies to validate PCR and standardized and validate qPCR are ongoing.

After ensuring that the drug was taken correctly, if the parasite is found to be persistent, it is necessary to take into account the possibility that it has developed resistance. Possible regional differences (host, T. cruzi strain, etc.), have been described as well; however, additional observations are required to confirm this hypothesis.

Even in cured patients, antibodies may remain detectable in sera for years after etiologic treatment until they become negative. Given this occurrence, it would be necessary to investigate the clinical history of reactive serology patients by asking, "Did he or she receive treatment in the past?" When the serological test yields an affirmative result, we must examine whether the reactivity is suggestive of an ongoing infection or if the patient is immune. been treated and is becoming negative.

The primary health care system is now responsible for the majority of diagnostic and treatment responsibilities under current recommendations. However, there are some fundamental limitations to the treatment of infected patients, but numerous studies are looking for solutions.

(Current medications are able to cure infection (or prevent disease) in adult patients during the chronic phase, which is when the majority of infected patients first come into contact. Clinical trials to demonstrate the effects of conventional treatment on this population are either finished or ongoing.

b) A new pediatric formulation of benznidazole is being tested for its ability to eradicate infection in infants and children who have recently developed a chronic infection. The majority of new cases involve congenital infections in newborns.

In general, the development of pediatric formulations and the development of new medications with shorter treatment durations and fewer adverse effects ought to be the top priorities in Chagas disease research. In the Clinical Trial for the Treatment of Chronic Chagas Disease with Posaconazole and Benznidazole, some strategies are being used, such as screening new compounds, testing drugs developed for other prescriptions like pozanonzole, or developing new compounds. Another way to look for new treatments is to look for compounds that have different ways of working together.

Every patient infected with T. cruzi must be (children) or should be treated (adults) according to current disease understanding during the chronic phase. The infection can be cured and the Chagas-related heart disease or cardiomyopathy can be reduced or prevented with treatment. Based on clinical and implementation research, the current benefits and drawbacks of etiological treatment serve to prioritize strategies in primary care, putting an emphasis on completing the treatment plan rather than demonstrating serological negativization.

Chapter 4

Various Treatment Options And Supplements For Quick Recovery From Chagas Disease

The most effective treatments seem to be natural ones because they don't harm the immune system or the gut like medications do.

Natural Chagas Disease Therapy
Bioenergetics In order to identify and get rid of the parasite, balancing as a natural treatment for Chagas disease involves exposing the body to its

electromagnetic signature. To aid in the body's correct and efficient defense against the illness, the immune system, detoxification processes, and cell and organ elimination can all be balanced. A parasite infection signifies that for some reason, the body is unable to attack and get rid of the invader as it should. By balance, the body's capacity for killing and detoxifying can be recovered.

Natural Anti-Parasitics

Natural acne treatments: Natural foods, herbs, and other products can be very effective against parasites.

Neem

Vidanga

Triphala

Olive leaf extracts

Raw

Garlic

Clove

Goldenseal

Pau d'arco

Oil of oregano

Rife Machine

Pumpkin seeds (pumpkin seed tea can be particularly effective) Utilizing electromagnetic frequencies to promote detoxification and kill specific parasites

Detoxification

When fighting an infection caused by a parasite or microorganism, the first and most crucial step is to open the pathways for elimination. A buildup of dead, toxic parasites that end up spilling into the blood and causing exasperated symptoms can occur if the lymphatic system, liver, and other eliminatory organs and pathways are clogged and you begin killing the parasites too quickly. Make sure your bowels are moving, that your lymphatic system is clear, and that your liver is supported. When you start to feel the effects of killing the parasites, you might want to slow down (up your dose) and do more detoxification.

Nutritional Therapy

It is essential to ensure that digestion is not hampered or compromised. Parasites have a feast to eat and thrive on if food is allowed to ferment in the intestines. It can be extremely beneficial to work with a holistic nutritionist to implement anti-parasitic foods and to restore and repair digestion and intestinal health.

Minimize or eliminate exposure to the environment, as well as foods that support parasite growth.

Alcohol

Coffee

Antibiotics

Eggs

Meat

Sugar

Whole grains

Refined foods

Processed foods and pork, which are frequently contaminated with parasites, birth control pills, toxins, and heavy metals are some of the parasite-fighting nutrients.

Omega 3 fatty acids

(positively influence the diversity of the gut flora), fiber (softens and plumps stool, ensures proper bowel movement for the elimination of parasites), glycine (regulates inflammation and improves enterocyte function in the intestinal tract), zinc (promotes enzymatic processes and strengthens the immune system to fight infection), and probiotics (to attack the bad intestinal critter while restoring good bacteria to the gut). Because parasites feed and thrive on heavy metals, toxins, and other pathogens, it is crucial to address heavy metal toxicity alongside parasite killing. Hence, overall detoxification is an essential component of parasite cleansing once more.

Tools for Heavy Metal Detoxification

Zeolite

Cilantro

Celery Juice

Spirulina & Chlorella

Conclusion

Chagas disease is an infection caused by a parasite called Trypanosoma cruzi. The most affected populations in Latin America are those who reside in rural areas. According to estimates, 300,000 People suffer from chagas sickness.

Chagas disease is an infection caused by a parasite called Trypanosome cruzi. This parasite is produced by an infected blood-sucking diatomite bug. Humans catch illnesses from insects. An infection develops when an infected bug's feces get into an open wound or mucous membrane, such as the nose or eyes. Moreover, the following things can transmit an infection

Ingesting tainted water typically in endemic or outbreak areas birth defect transmission (from mother to child) transfusions of blood transplantation of organs ingesting tainted water Once infected, it is typical for people to exhibit minimal or no symptoms, leaving them ignorant of their infection. Rarely, a life-threatening illness may strike an infected person in the days or weeks after infection. Years or even decades after the illness, which may linger for years, some patients get severe heart or digestive problems.

Late or chronic phase: can last for years or decades. In the beginning, mild symptoms like fever, body aches, tiredness, and swelling around where the parasite entered the body can occur. Although the initial stage of the disease can be fatal in rare instances, most people do not experience any health issues once they become infected.

About one-third of patients experience serious heart or gastrointestinal issues in the late phase. Heart disease can cause sudden death and is common in the chronic phase. Serious diseases are more likely to strike those with immune disorders, such as HIV/AIDS patients or recipients of organ transplants.

Alternatives to Therapy The first Chagas disease treatment to receive approval in the US was benznidazole. Between the ages of 2 and 12, children with Chagas disease should take benznidazole.

The most frequent negative effects of taking benznidazole were nausea, vomiting, headaches, abnormal white blood cell counts, urticaria (hives), pruritus (itching), and decreased appetite.

Pregnant women should not use benznidazole as it could harm the developing fetus.

www.ingramcontent.com/pod-product-compliance
Lightning Source LLC
Chambersburg PA
CBHW050752250726
48662CB00005B/2174